The
CELERY JUiCE
SOLUTION
Recipe Book

The CELERY JUiCE SOLUTION Recipe Book

HARNESS THE AMAZING BENEFITS OF CELERY WITH OVER 75+ HEALTH BOOSTING CELERY JUICE & GREEN SMOOTHIE RECIPES

DISCLAIMER

CONTENTS

DIGESTIVE HEALTH SMOOTHIES

ENERGY BOOST SMOOTHIES

SMOOTHIES FOR SKIN

CLEAN & GREEN SMOOTHIES

SUPERFOOD SMOOTHIES

INTRODUCTION

Celery juice is being hailed as a miracle cure for a growing list of ailments and illnesses.

The growing global movement promoting celery juice is reaching dizzying heights, with a rising list of celebrities including Gwyneth Paltrow, Pharrell Williams and Elle Macpherson endorsing its benefits.

The celery wellness trend has benefitted from the increasing knowledge about the harmful effects of sugar intake, as well as also the (sometimes unfair or inaccurate) negative press surrounding carbs. Celery is very low in both sugar and carbs, so those who have may have shunned juicing with fruit due to its potentially high sugar content have now found favour with this green veggie wonder.

The power of social media, in particular Instagram, has helped fuel the rapid growth in the popularity of celery juice, but what exactly are the benefits of this 'miracle worker'?

BENEFITS OF CELERY JUICE

Raw celery juice is packed with an array of nutrients including essential vitamins, minerals and antioxidants critical to regular and optimal bodily function.

AIDS WEIGHT LOSS

The average celery stick contains just 6 calories. Drinking celery juice is a great option when aiming to lose weight. It is filling, so helps combat cravings and keep your appetite in check.

GREAT FOR SKIN

Celery is made up 95% water, so when consumed regularly it can help to keep skin hydrated and supple. The antioxidant properties of celery help to neutralise harmful free radicals, removing toxins, therefore purifying skin and making it appear clearer. Vitamins A, B, C, K, niacin and folate, which are all present in celery, help to repair damaged skin and promote new cell growth and glowing skin.

CANCER PREVENTION

Research suggests that the flavonoids (plant pigments) found in celery may help prevent the growth of cancer, as well as the onset of cardiovascular disease and cognitive impairment.

LOWER CHOLESTEROL AND BLOOD PRESSURE

One of the chemical constituents of celery is butylphthalide, which is responsible for its smell and taste. Studies suggest that butylphthalide may help in reducing the levels of bad cholesterol in our blood stream and, by relaxing the muscles around our blood vessels and reducing stress hormones, it can help control blood pressure.

DIGESTIVE HEALTH

Due to its antioxidant and anti-inflammatory nutrients, celery promotes digestive health and can help improve stomach lining health. The presence of soluble and insoluble fibre promotes general gut health.

HAIR

The same vitamins are also great for hair, nourishing roots, keeping the scalp hydrated and stimulating hair growth.

BLADDER HEALTH

The high level of water content in celery facilitates the production of urine and helps us stay healthy. The urinary system eliminates waste from the body after it is filtered through the kidney then stored in the bladder. Urination regulates blood volume and blood pressure.

ACID BALANCE

Celery has a very low level of acidity. Drinking celery juice can help regulate and stabilize the PH levels in your body and stop the build up of acid; particularly helpful if you suffer from conditions such as acid reflux.

ANTI-INFLAMMATORY PROPERTIES

The highly anti-inflammatory elements of celery can help with inflammation in bone diseases such as arthritis, as well as respiratory conditions like bronchitis and asthma.

AIDS SLEEP

Celery contains magnesium, which is known to relax nerves and can aid sleep.

The benefits of drinking celery juice are vast and so too are the multitude of different ways your daily intake can be prepared.

The simplest, and arguably most effective way, to benefit from the healing properties of celery juice is to consume it in its purest form.

Take approx 8 organic celery sticks, remove the leaves and rinse.
Run the celery through a juicer and drink immediately (approx. 400ml)
Alternatively you can use a high-powered blender and if you wish, strain through a mesh strainer or cheesecloth to remove any pulp.

Consume daily, first thing in the morning, on an empty stomach.

It is important to remember that while there are many potential health benefits of drinking celery juice, it should not be used as a replacement for a balanced diet. Instead, it should form part of a portfolio of whole foods consumed daily – protein, carbohydrates and fats with a variety of fresh vegetables. This will ensure you don't miss out on the unique nutrients that other whole foods and vegetables can provide.

Drinking pure celery juice can take a little getting used to as it is not to everyone's taste. If you can't drink a full glass each morning, try having just half a glass and gradually increasing the amount you have each day. Some people experiment taking the 'edge' off the taste by adding cucumber or apple. This daily dose of a glass of celery juice should help you see the health benefits you are seeking.

With celery now a natural part of your morning routine, you'll be able to use our delicious range of refreshing celery juices and smoothie ideas as an additional nutrient boost at any time of the day. Each of our simple and tasty recipes all pack a punch of celery and super foods, which will help to keep your celery content fresh and interesting whilst still delivering the healing powers every day of the week.

This book is packed with delicious and simple green smoothies and juices. It's so easy to make a green smoothie for a snack or breakfast, and the energy and nutrient boost you receive really is palpable. All our juices and smoothies can be made in a high-powered blender, such as a Nutribullet, or in a juicer if you prefer. It is not essential to strain our celery drinks - some prefer to do this to make it quicker to drink and absorb, but it's really a personal preference.

To help make your celery drinks fuss-free, follow these quick tips;

- Prepare your shopping list. Take some time to select which drinks you want to prepare in advance. As with all food shopping, make a note of all the ingredients and quantities you need. Depending on the ingredients, it's best not to shop too far in advance to ensure you are getting the freshest produce available.
- We recommend buying organic produce whenever you can (if your budget allows). Organic produce can give a better yield and flavour. Remember, almost all fruit can be frozen.
- Wash your fruit and veg before juicing. This needn't take up much time, but all produce should be washed clean of any traces of bacteria, pesticides and insects.
- To save time, prepare produce the night before for early morning drinks.
- Cut up any produce that may not fit into the cup of your blender, but only do this just before juicing to keep it as fresh as possible.
- Wash your blender/juicer parts immediately after use. As tempting as it may be to leave until a little later, you'll be glad you took the few minutes to rinse and wash before any residue has hardened.
- Substitute where you need. If you can't source a particular ingredient, try another instead. More often than not you will find the use of a different fruit or veg makes a really interesting and delicious alternative. In our recipes we offer some advice on alternatives, but have the confidence to choose your own too!
- Some smoothies and juices are sweeter than others. Try drinking these with a straw, you'll find them easier to drink and enjoy.
- Drink lots of water!

As with any food, there is a risk of sensitivity that might cause allergic reactions. Celery can be known to cause reactions such as itchiness or mild swelling of the mouth. If you have previously suffered from a food allergy, or are taking medication or supplements, we advise that you consult with a health professional before drinking celery juice.

Welcome to the exciting new world of celery juice and its health benefits. Enjoy!

GREEN BREAKFAST SMOOTHIES

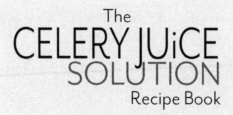

The
CELERY JUiCE
SOLUTION
Recipe Book

GRAPE, SPINACH & COCONUT SMOOTHIE

Ingredients

RICH IN FIBRE

- 2 celery stalks, chopped
- 1 handful seedless green grapes
- 1 handful spinach
- 200ml/7floz light coconut milk
- Handful of ice cubes

Method

1 Rinse the celery, grapes and the spinach well. Remove any thick stalks from the spinach.

2 Add all the ingredients to the blender, making sure they do not go past the MAX line on your machine.

3 Use just a few ice cubes to start with, until you get the desired consistency.

4 Blend until smooth.

CHEF'S NOTE
In Sanskrit, the coconut palm is known as kalpa vriksha - 'tree which gives all that is necessary for living'.

COCONUT GREEN SMOOTHIE

Ingredients

- 175ml/6floz coconut water
- 60ml/2floz coconut milk
- 1 tbsp ground flax seeds
- ½ lemon
- ¼ apple

- ¼ orange
- 2 stalks of celery, chopped
- Handful of kale
- 3 romaine lettuce leaves

Method

1 Rinse the celery, kale and lettuce. Roughly chop and remove any thick stalks from the kale.

2 Peel and de-seed the lemon and orange. Core the apple.

3 Add all the ingredients to the blender, making sure they do not go past the MAX line on your machine.

4 Blend until smooth.

CHEF'S NOTE
Flax seeds are thought to help improve digestion, promote clear skin, lower cholesterol & reduce sugar cravings.

GREEN HONEY MANGO SMOOTHIE

Ingredients

ALKALI RESERVES

- ½ ripe mango
- 1 handful spinach
- 2 celery stalks, chopped
- 200ml/7 floz light coconut milk
- 2 tbsp plain low-fat yogurt
- 1 tbsp honey

Method

1 Peel and stone the mango.

2 Wash the celery & spinach..

3 Add all the ingredients to the blender, making sure they do not go past the MAX line on your machine.

4 Blend until smooth.

CHEF'S NOTE

Great for breakfast smoothies, low-fat yogurt is not only low in calories, but it also has plenty of beneficial nutrients and probiotics that can boost your overall health.

BLUEBERRY BREAKFAST

Ingredients

BLUEBERRY POWER →

- 1 tbsp oats
- 2 handfuls spinach
- 60g/2½oz fresh blueberries
- 200ml/7floz unsweetened almond milk
- 1 tsp agave nectar or honey
- ½-1 tsp grated fresh ginger root
- 2 celery stalks, chopped

Method

1 Place the oats in a little water in the blender and soak until they have softened (about 15 minutes).

2 Rinse the blueberries, spinach and celery. Remove any the stalks from the spinach.

3 Add them and the other ingredients to the softened oats, making sure they do not go past the MAX line on your machine (add extra water if you like).

4 Blend until smooth.

CHEF'S NOTE
Soya milk is also good with this lovely breakfast smoothie. For extra morning energy try adding half a banana.

NUTMEG PUMPKIN SMOOTHIE

Ingredients

VITAMIN A +

- 200ml/7 floz unsweetened almond milk
- 200g/7oz fresh pumpkin flesh
- 1 handful shredded greens
- 2 celery stalks, chopped
- 1 tbsp honey
- ¼ tsp ground nutmeg
- Water

Method

1 Peel and de-seed the pumpkin.

2 Rinse the shredded greens and celery.

3 Add all the ingredients to the blender, making sure they do not go past the MAX line on your machine.

4 Use as much or as little water as you wish to get the consistency you prefer. For a thicker smoothie don't add any at all.

CHEF'S NOTE
Nutmeg contains antioxidants and disease-preventing phytochemicals, some of which are completely unique.

DATE SMOOTHIE

Ingredients

VITAMIN B+

- 175ml/6floz light coconut milk
- 1 handful pitted dates
- 1 handful spinach
- 1 handful kale
- 2 celery stalks, chopped
- Handful of ice cubes

Method

1 Rinse the spinach, kale & celery well. Remove any thick stalks from the spinach.

2 Add all the ingredients to the blender, making sure they do not go past the MAX line on your machine (use as many of the ice cubes as you wish).

3 Blend until smooth.

CHEF'S NOTE
Fibre rich, dates are easily digested, allowing your body to make full use of their goodness.

KALE, BANANA & PINEAPPLE SMOOTHIE

Ingredients

NUTRIENT DENSE

- 120ml/4 floz light coconut milk
- 1 handful kale
- 2 celery stalks, chopped
- ¼ pineapple
- 1 banana

Method

1 Rinse the kale and remove any thick stalks.

2 Rinse the celery.

3 Peel and roughly chop the fresh pineapple.

4 Peel the banana and break into three pieces.

5 Add all the ingredients to the blender, making sure they do not go past the MAX line on your machine.

6 Blend until smooth.

CHEF'S NOTE
Feel free to add more coconut milk or water to create your desired consistency.

SWEET SPINACH & BANANA SMOOTHIE

Ingredients

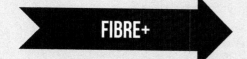

- 2 handfuls spinach
- 1 banana
- 2 celery stalks, chopped
- 1 carrot
- 4 tbsp low fat natural yogurt
- 1 tbsp honey
- Handful of ice cubes

Method

1 Rinse the spinach, celery and the carrot well. Roughly chop the carrot and remove any thick stalks from the spinach.

2 Peel the banana and break into three pieces.

3 Add all the ingredients to the blender, making sure they do not go past the MAX line on your machine.

4 Blend until smooth.

CHEF'S NOTE
Add more yoghurt to suit your own taste, making sure you keep below the MAX line.

AVOCADO, BANANA & KIWI SMOOTHIE

Ingredients

CREAMY!

- 1 handful spinach
- ½ avocado
- 1 banana
- 1 kiwi
- 300ml/10½floz almond milk
- ¼ tsp ground cinnamon
- 2 celery stalks, chopped

Method

1 Rinse the celery & spinach then remove any thick stalks.

2 Halve, stone and peel the avocado. Peel the banana and break into three pieces.

3 Peel the kiwi and halve.

4 Add all the ingredients to the blender, making sure they do not go past the MAX line on your machine.

5 Blend until smooth.

CHEF'S NOTE
Kiwi is also one of the few foods rich in vitamin B6, which supports the immune system.

CLEMENTINE & SPINACH CHIA SMOOTHIE

Ingredients

LACTOSE FREE

- 1 handful spinach
- 3 seedless clementines
- 1 banana
- 120ml/4floz soya milk
- 1 tbsp chai seeds
- 1 celery stalk, chopped

Method

1 Rinse the celery & spinach well, removing any thick stalks from the spinach.

2 Peel the clementines. Peel the banana and break into three pieces.

3 Add all the ingredients to the blender, making sure they do not go past the MAX line on your machine.

4 Blend until smooth.

CHEF'S NOTE
A little added organic honey or agave nectar makes this breakfast smoothie a sweet treat.

BLUEBERRY BLAST

Ingredients

- 1 handful fresh blueberries
- 1 celery stalk, chopped
- 1 handful spinach
- 1 banana
- ½ carrot
- ½ lemon
- 1 tbsp flax seeds
- Water

Method

1 Wash the blueberries, celery & spinach.

2 Wash, top & tail the carrot.

3 Remove any thick stalks from the spinach.

4 Peel the banana and break into three pieces.

5 Add all the ingredients to the blender, making sure they do not go past the MAX line on your machine.

6 Blend until smooth.

CHEF'S NOTE

The high fibre, antioxidant and anti-inflammatory content of flaxseed are great for healthy smoothies.

ALMOND BUTTER VANILLA SMOOTHIE

Ingredients

- 1 pear
- 1 celery stalk, chopped
- 200ml/7floz unsweetened almond milk
- 1 handful spinach
- 2 tbsp oats
- 1 tbsp almond butter
- ¼ tsp vanilla extract
- Handful of ice cubes

Method

1 Rinse the celery, spinach and pear.

2 Core the pear and remove any thick stalks from the spinach.

3 Add all the ingredients to the blender, making sure they do not go past the MAX line on your machine.

4 Blend until smooth.

CHEF'S NOTE
Packed with goodness, this breakfast smoothie will slowly release energy throughout the morning to help keep you energised.

STRAWBERRY & ALMOND BUTTER SMOOTHIE

Ingredients

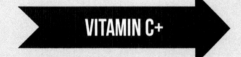

- 200ml/7floz almond milk
- 4 strawberries
- ½ banana
- 2 handfuls shredded greens
- 1 tbsp flax seeds
- 1 tbsp almond butter
- 2 celery stalks, chopped

Method

1 Rinse the strawberries, celery and greens.

2 Peel the banana.

3 Add all the ingredients to the blender, making sure they do not go past the MAX line on your machine.

4 Blend until smooth.

CHEF'S NOTE
Add more strawberries to suit your taste, or try a handful of raspberries too.

DETOX & CLEANSE SMOOTHIES

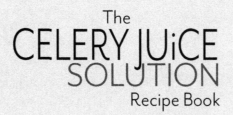

The
CELERY JUiCE
SOLUTION
Recipe Book

SUPER-CLEANSING SMOOTHIE

Ingredients

- 1 handful spinach
- 1 Romaine lettuce
- ¼ cucumber
- 1 celery stalk, chopped
- 1 pear
- 1 banana

- 250ml/8 floz coconut water
- 4 fresh mint leaves
- ½ lemon
- 1 tbsp chia seeds
- 1cm/½ inch fresh ginger root, peeled

Method

1 Rinse the ingredients well.

2 Core the pear. Peel the banana. Peel and de-seed the lemon.

3 Add all the ingredients to the blender, making sure they do not go past the MAX line on your machine.

4 Blend until smooth.

CHEF'S NOTE
Spice it up with a pinch of cayenne pepper, cinnamon and turmeric.

GRAPEFRUIT & SPINACH SMOOTHIE

Ingredients

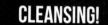

CLEANSING!

- 1 grapefruit
- 1 handful seedless green grapes
- ½ banana
- 1 handful spinach
- 1cm/½ inch fresh ginger root, peeled
- 1 date
- 2 celery stalks, chopped

Method

1 Rinse the grapes, celery and the spinach well; remove any thick stalks from the spinach

2 Peel and de-seed the grapefruit. Peel the banana and stone the date.

3 Add all the ingredients to the blender, making sure they do not go past the MAX line on your machine.

4 Blend until smooth.

CHEF'S NOTE
The date will add a subtle natural sweetness to this smoothie.

APPLE & KALE SMOOTHIE

SERVES 1

Ingredients

DIETARY FIBRE

- 1 handful kale
- 1 apple
- 2 celery stalks, chopped
- 250ml/8½ floz coconut water
- Handful of ice cubes

Method

1 Rinse the kale, celery and the apple well.

2 Remove any thick stalks from the kale and core the apple

3 Add all the ingredients to the blender, making sure they do not go past the MAX line on your machine.

4 Blend until smooth.

CHEF'S NOTE
Kale is packed with fibre and sulphur, both great for detoxifying your body and keeping your liver healthy.

SIMPLE SPINACH & SPICE SMOOTHIE

Ingredients

HEALING!

- 2cm/1 inch fresh ginger root
- ½ - 1 tsp ground cinnamon
- 2 handfuls spinach
- 2 celery stalks, chopped
- Water

Method

1 Rinse the spinach well and remove any thick stalks.

2 Peel and grate the ginger.

3 Add all the ingredients to the blender, making sure they do not go past the MAX line on your machine.

4 Blend until smooth.

CHEF'S NOTE
Ginger is thought to cleanse the body by stimulating digestion, circulation and sweating.

PEAR & GINGER FLAX SMOOTHIE

Ingredients

NATURALLY SWEET!

- 1 pear
- 1 handful spinach
- 1 tbsp flax seeds
- 1 tsp coconut oil
- 2cm/1 inch fresh ginger root
- 2 tsp honey
- 2 celery stalks, chopped

Method

1 Rinse the pear, celery and the spinach, then remove any thick stalks from the spinach.

2 Core the pear. Peel & grate the ginger.

3 Add all the ingredients to the blender, making sure they do not go past the MAX line on your machine.

4 Blend until smooth.

CHEF'S NOTE
Flax seeds are thought to help eliminate the toxins from the body, normalise the metabolism, reduce blood sugar levels and regulate appetite.

GREEN & FRUITY JUICE

SERVES 1

Ingredients

- ¼ cucumber
- 1 handful spinach
- ½ avocado
- 1 celery stalk, chopped

- 2 sprigs mint
- 1 kiwi
- ½ apple
- Water

Method

1 Rinse the ingredients well and remove any thick stalks from the spinach.

2 Halve, stone & peel the avocado. Peel the kiwi fruit. Core the apple.

3 Add all the ingredients to the blender, making sure they do not go past the MAX line on your machine.

4 Blend until smooth.

CHEF'S NOTE
Raw spinach is rich in glutathione, which is helpful to overall well-being.

SPINACH, MINT & GINGER JUICE

Ingredients

HYDRATING!

- 1 handful spinach
- 1 handful fresh mint
- 1 tbsp lemon juice
- ½ cucumber
- 4 celery stalks, chopped
- 2cm/1 inch fresh ginger root
- Water

Method

1 Rinse the ingredients well and remove any thick stalks from the spinach.

2 Peel and grate the ginger.

3 Add all the ingredients to the blender, making sure they do not go past the MAX line on your machine.

4 Blend until smooth.

CHEF'S NOTE
The hydrating properties of cucumber, along with the lemon juice, create a cleansing effect that helps to clear out the digestive system.

WINTER SMOOTHIE

SERVES 1

Ingredients

- 1 apple
- 1 pear
- 1 handful fresh cranberries
- 2cm/1 inch fresh ginger root

- 3 large kale leaves
- 1 handful shredded green cabbage
- 1 celery stalk, chopped

Method

1 Wash the ingredients well.

2 Core the apple and pear. Peel and grate the ginger.

3 Add all the ingredients to the blender, making sure they do not go past the MAX line on your machine.

4 Blend until smooth.

CHEF'S NOTE

There is some evidence that links cranberries to a reduced risk of kidney stones, cardiovascular disease and cancer.

CARROT, PEAR & BROCCOLI SMOOTHIE

Ingredients

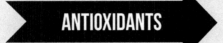

- 1 carrot
- ½ pear
- 2 celery stalks, chopped
- 200g/7oz broccoli florets
- Water

Method

1 Rinse the ingredients well.

2 Core the pear. Nip the ends off the carrot.

3 Add all the ingredients to the blender, making sure they do not go past the MAX line on your machine.

4 Blend until smooth.

CHEF'S NOTE
Broccoli has a number of outstanding health properties, including high concentrations of essential vitamins & fibre.

DIGESTIVE HEALTH SMOOTHIES

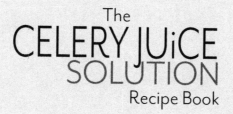

The
CELERY JUiCE
SOLUTION
Recipe Book

PINEAPPLE & PARSLEY SMOOTHIE

Ingredients

- ½ fresh pineapple
- ½ banana
- 120ml/4 floz water
- 120ml/4 floz coconut water
- A few sprigs fresh parsley

- 1 celery stalk, chopped
- 1 handful spinach
- ¼ avocado
- 1 tsp freshly grated ginger root

Method

1 Pour the water and coconut water into the blender.

2 Peel the pineapple & banana and add to the cup.

3 Peel and stone the avocado. Give the parsley and spinach a rinse, and add to blender, along with the grated ginger, making sure they do not go past the MAX line on your machine.

4 Blend until smooth.

CHEF'S NOTE
Ginger helps improve digestion, prevents bloating and decreases intestinal gas.

CORIANDER & GINGER SMOOTHIE

Ingredients

- 1 handful fresh coriander
- 1 cucumber
- 3 tbsp lime juice
- 1-inch peeled fresh ginger root
- ¼ fresh pineapple
- 1 tomato
- 1 celery stalk, chopped

Method

1 Rinse the coriander, cucumber, celery and tomato.

2 Roughly chop the cucumber, halve the tomato and peel the pineapple.

3 Add all the ingredients to the blender, making sure they do not go past the MAX line on your machine.

4 Blend until smooth.

CHEF'S NOTE
Coriander has been used to treat stomach disorders in traditional Chinese medicine throughout the ages.

BLUEBERRY & SPINACH SMOOTHIE

Ingredients

DIGESTION BOOSTER

- 1 handful blueberries
- 2 handfuls spinach
- ½ tbsp ground flax seeds
- 120ml/½ cup coconut milk
- 1 celery stalk, chopped

Method

1 Rinse the blueberries, celery and the spinach well.

2 Add all the ingredients to the blender, making sure they do not go past the MAX line on your machine. Add a little water if needed to take it to the line (or a little more coconut water)

3 Blend until smooth.

CHEF'S NOTE
Ground flax seeds are a good source of soluble fibre, which is essential to aid healthy digestion.

SOOTHING GREEN FRUIT SMOOTHIE

Ingredients

- 1 handful shredded Romaine, or green leaf lettuce
- 1 handful spinach
- 1 slice of fennel bulb
- ¼ apple
- ¼ pear
- 1 small handful fresh mint
- 1 small handful fresh coriander
- 1 tbsp lemon juice
- 1 celery stalk, chopped

Method

1 Rinse the ingredients well.

2 Remove any thick stalks from the spinach. Core the apple and pear,

3 Add all the ingredients to the blender, making sure they do not go past the MAX line on your machine.

4 Blend until smooth.

CHEF'S NOTE

In Germany, coriander is officially approved for the treatment of mild gastrointestinal upsets, and to help stimulate the appetite.

CABBAGE, PINEAPPLE & PAPAYA SMOOTHIE

SERVES 1

Ingredients

TOXIN CLEANSER

- ¼ pineapple
- ¼ papaya
- 1 handful shredded cabbage
- 1 handful spinach
- 200ml/7floz coconut water
- 1 celery stalk, chopped

Method

1 Wash the cabbage & spinach.

2 Peel the pineapple & papaya (don't worry about the seeds if you have a powerful blender).

3 Add all the ingredients to the blender, making sure they do not go past the MAX line on your machine.

4 Blend until smooth.

CHEF'S NOTE
Coconut water is thought to aid digestion by helping to eliminate body waste and release toxins.

GREEN CHIA SMOOTHIE

Ingredients

- 2 tbsp natural Greek yoghurt
- 1 handful spinach
- 1 handful kale
- 2 tbsp chia seeds
- 1 celery stalk, chopped
- ½ cucumber
- ½ apple
- 1 tbsp lemon juice
- A few fresh mint leaves

Method

1 Rinse the spinach, celery, kale, cucumber, apple and mint.

2 Roughly chop the cucumber, core the apple and remove any thick stalks from the spinach & kale.

3 Add all the ingredients to the blender, making sure they do not go past the MAX line on your machine.

4 Blend until smooth.

CHEF'S NOTE
The ancient Aztecs long promoted the health benefits of chia seeds as a remedy for constipation.

FRUIT & GINGER SMOOTHIE

SERVES 1

Ingredients

PROTEIN RICH

- 1 handful shredded greens
- ½ avocado
- ½ banana
- 1 inch/2cm piece fresh ginger root
- 200g/7oz pineapple
- 240ml/8floz coconut water
- 1 celery stalk, chopped

Method

1 Rinse the greens and remove any thick stalks.

2 Pour the coconut water and celery into the blender.

3 Halve, stone and peel the avocado. Peel the banana, ginger root and pineapple and add to the cup, making sure they do not go past the MAX line on your machine.

4 Blend until smooth.

CHEF'S NOTE
The fibre content of green vegetables makes them a natural choice for digestive system support.

GREEN KEFIR SMOOTHIE

Ingredients

PROBIOTICS

- 360ml/12½floz coconut water kefir
- 1 handful fresh pea shoots
- 1 handful fresh spinach
- 1 celery stalk
- 1 carrot

Method

1 Rinse the ingredients well.

2 Remove any thick stalks from the spinach and nip the ends off the carrot.

3 Add all the ingredients to the blender, making sure they do not go past the MAX line on your machine.

4 Blend until smooth.

CHEF'S NOTE

Coconut water kefir is a naturally fermented beverage made from young coconuts. If you can't buy kefir just use regular coconut water.

CABBAGE & HONEY SMOOTHIE

Ingredients

AIDS DIGESTION

- 2 handfuls shredded green cabbage
- 2 tbsp lemon juice
- 1 tbsp organic honey
- 2 celery stalks, chopped
- Water

Method

1 Rinse the cabbage and celery well and put them in the blender.

2 Add the rest of the ingredients, making sure they don't go past the MAX line on your machine.

3 Blend until smooth.

CHEF'S NOTE
This smoothie is good for general intestinal health. Drink twice a day to combat constipation problems.

FRUITY HEMP SMOOTHIE

Ingredients

- 1 banana
- 1 handful strawberries
- 1 handful spinach
- 2 tbsp hulled hemp seeds
- 1 tbsp pea protein powder
- 200ml/7 floz coconut water
- 1 tsp agave nectar
- 1 celery stalk, chopped

Method

1 Peel the banana and break into three pieces.

2 Rinse the spinach, celery and strawberries well.

3 Add all the ingredients to the blender, making sure they do not go past the MAX line on your machine.

4 Blend until smooth.

CHEF'S NOTE

Hemp seeds aid digestion, balance hormones and improve metabolism.

SOYA KIWI SMOOTHIE

Ingredients

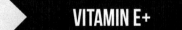

VITAMIN E+

- 1 handful kale
- 2 celery stalks, chopped
- 1 pear
- 2 kiwi fruits
- 200ml/7floz soya milk

Method

1 Rinse the kale, celery and pear.

2 Core the pear and peel the kiwi fruits.

3 Add all the ingredients to the blender, making sure they do not go past the MAX line on your machine.

4 Blend until smooth.

CHEF'S NOTE
Kiwis are believed to contain a unique compound which helps to digest the proteins found in red meat.

ENERGY BOOST SMOOTHIES

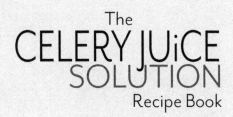

The
CELERY JUiCE
SOLUTION
Recipe Book

MATCHA AND PEAR SMOOTHIE

Ingredients

ANTIOXIDANTS

- 1 handful spinach
- 1 pear
- ½ tsp matcha green tea powder
- 300ml/10½ floz unsweetened almond milk
- 1 celery stalk, chopped

Method

1 Rinse the spinach, celery and pear. Core the pear and remove any hard stalks from the spinach.

2 Add all the ingredients to the blender, making sure they do not go past the MAX line on your machine.

3 Add a little more water if needed.

4 Blend until smooth.

CHEF'S NOTE
Matcha is powdered green tea leaves. Because whole leaves are ingested, it's a more potent source of goodness than steeped green tea.

GREEN AVOCADO & COCONUT SMOOTHIE

Ingredients

- ½ avocado
- 1 handful kale
- ½ apple
- 1 handful spinach

- 250ml/8½ floz coconut water
- 4 fresh mint leaves
- 1 celery stalk, chopped
- Water

Method

1 Wash the kale, celery, spinach, mint and apple. Cut any thick stems from the kale and spinach.

2 Core the apple. Peel and stone the avocado.

3 Add all the ingredients to the blender, making sure they do not go past the MAX line on your machine.

4 Add a little more water if needed.

5 Blend until smooth.

CHEF'S NOTE

Avocados are rich in monosaturated fats. These are good fats that your body uses to create energy quickly.

GREEN FRUIT SMOOTHIE

Ingredients

NUTRIENT DENSE

- ½ cucumber
- 1 stalk celery, chopped
- 1 handful kale
- 1 apple
- 1 pear
- 1 tsp lemon juice
- Water

Method

1 Rinse the ingredients well.

2 Core the apple and pear. Remove any thick stalks from the kale.

3 Add all the ingredients to the blender, making sure they do not go past the MAX line on your machine.

4 Add a little water if needed.

5 Blend until smooth.

CHEF'S NOTE
Kale is a real energy booster that provides the essential minerals of copper, potassium, iron and phosphorus.

ORANGE AND SPINACH SMOOTHIE

Ingredients

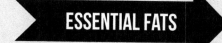

- 1 orange
- ½ banana
- 1 handful spinach
- 120ml/4floz coconut water
- 1 tbsp hemp seeds
- 1 celery stalk, chopped

Method

1 Rinse the spinach and remove any thick stalks.

2 Peel and de-seed the orange.

3 Peel the banana.

4 Add all the ingredients to the blender, making sure they do not go past the MAX line on your machine.

5 Add a little more water if needed.

6 Blend until smooth.

CHEF'S NOTE
Containing essential omega-3 fats, hemp seeds provide long sustaining energy.

APPLE & SPINACH SMOOTHIE

Ingredients

ENERGY BOOST

- 2 apples
- 1 handful seedless green grapes
- 1 handful spinach
- 1 kiwi
- 2 celery stalks, chopped
- Water

Method

1 Rinse the apples, grapes, spinach and celery.

2 Core the apples.

3 Peel the kiwi fruit and cut it in two.

4 Add all the ingredients to the blender, making sure they do not go past the MAX line on your machine.

5 Add a little water if needed.

6 Blend until smooth.

CHEF'S NOTE
Spinach is extremely high in magnesium and plays a vital role in producing energy.

LEMON GREEN BLAST

SERVES 1

Ingredients

- 5 celery stalks, chopped
- 1 handful of kale
- 1 handful of spinach
- 1 handful flat-leaf parsley
- 1 lemon
- 1 cucumber
- Water

Method

1 Rinse the ingredients well.

2 Remove any thick stalks from the kale and spinach.

3 Peel and de-seed the lemon. Roughly chop the cucumber.

4 Add all the ingredients to the blender, making sure they do not go past the MAX line on your machine.

5 Add a little water if needed.

6 Blend until smooth.

CHEF'S NOTE

Parsley contains lots of vitamin C that boosts cell regeneration and helps the body stay energised.

COCONUT & FLAX SMOOTHIE

SERVES 1

Ingredients

GOOD FATS

- 250ml/8½floz coconut water
- ½ pear
- ½ avocado
- 1 handful spinach
- 1 tbsp flax seeds
- 1 celery stalk, chopped

Method

1 Wash the pear, spinach & celery.

2 Remove any thick stalks from the spinach and core the pear.

3 Peel and stone the avocado.

4 Add all the ingredients to the blender, making sure they do not go past the MAX line on your machine.

5 Add a little more water if needed.

6 Blend until smooth.

CHEF'S NOTE
Flax seeds are one of the richest sources of vital Omega-3 fatty acids.

SPINACH & STRAWBERRY SMOOTHIE

Ingredients

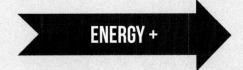

ENERGY +

- 2 handfuls spinach
- 1 apple
- 1 banana
- 5 strawberries
- ½ orange
- 2 celery stalk, chopped

Method

1 Rinse the spinach, celery, apple and strawberries.

2 Core the apple. Peel the banana and break into three pieces.

3 Peel and de-seed the orange.

4 Add all the ingredients to the blender, making sure they do not go past the MAX line on your machine.

5 Blend until smooth.

CHEF'S NOTE
Bananas boost energy by slowly releasing carbs into the bloodstream as glucose.

SPICED PERSIMMON SMOOTHIE

Ingredients

VITAMIN RICH

- 250ml/8½floz almond milk
- 1 persimmon
- 1 handful spinach
- ½ tsp cinnamon
- ¼ tsp cardamom
- 1 date
- 1 celery stalk, chopped

Method

1 Wash the persimmon, celery and the spinach. Cut the persimmon into quarters.

2 Halve and stone the date. Remove any thick stalks from the spinach.

3 Add all the ingredients to the blender, making sure they do not go past the MAX line on your machine.

4 Blend until smooth.

CHEF'S NOTE
Persimmons have a high vitamin and mineral content including vitamins A, C, E and B6, as well as dietary fibre, manganese, copper, magnesium, potassium, and phosphorous.

SWEET & SPICY GREEN SMOOTHIE

Ingredients

- 1 handful kale
- 1 apple
- ½ lemon
- 2cm/1 inch slice peeled, fresh ginger root

- ¼ tsp cayenne pepper
- 1 tbsp organic honey
- 1 celery stalk, chopped

Method

1 Rinse the kale, celery and apple.

2 Remove any thick stalks from the kale. Core the apple. Peel and de-seed the lemon.

3 Add all the ingredients to the blender, making sure they do not go past the MAX line on your machine.

4 Blend until smooth.

CHEF'S NOTE

Eating 'good carbs', such as honey, during a workout helps your muscles stay nourished longer and delays fatigue.

KALE & KIWI BLAST

Ingredients

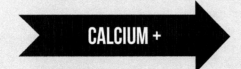

- 2 handfuls kale
- 2 kiwis
- 1 orange
- 2 tsp lemon juice
- 1 celery stalk, chopped

Method

1 Rinse the kale and remove any thick stalks

2 Peel the kiwi fruits and cut them in half.

3 Peel and de-seed the orange.

4 Add all the ingredients to the blender, making sure they do not go past the MAX line on your machine.

5 Blend until smooth.

CHEF'S NOTE
High in vitamins and minerals, kale is a great energy booster and a key source of calcium.

SMOOTHIES FOR SKIN

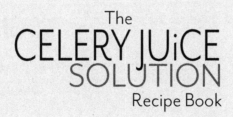

The
CELERY JUiCE
SOLUTION
Recipe Book

SWISS CHARD & GRAPE SMOOTHIE

Ingredients

- 2 handfuls Swiss chard
- 1 handful green seedless grapes
- 1 pear
- 1 orange
- 2 bananas
- 1 tsp chia seeds
- 1 celery stalk, chopped
- Ice

Method

1 Rinse the fruit and vegetables well.

2 Remove the stems from the chard and roughly chop the leaves.

3 Core the pear. Peel and de-seed the orange. Peel the bananas and break each one into three pieces.

4 Add all the ingredients to the blender, making sure they do not go past the MAX line on your machine.

5 Blend until smooth.

CHEF'S NOTE
The antioxidants in grapes can help increase blood circulation, leading to healthy and glowing skin.

ALMOND KALE SMOOTHIE

Ingredients

CLEANSING

- 250ml/8½floz unsweetened almond milk
- 1 handful kale leaves
- 1 banana
- 1 tbsp natural peanut butter
- 1 celery stalk, chopped

Method

1 Rinse the kale and cut off any thick stalks.

2 Peel the banana and break into three pieces.

3 Add all the ingredients to the blender, making sure they do not go past the MAX line on your machine.

4 Blend until smooth.

CHEF'S NOTE
The sulphur and fibre in kale aids body detoxification.

PROTEIN BLAST

Ingredients

PROTEIN+

- 120ml/4floz coconut water
- 2 handfuls kale
- 300g/11oz fresh pineapple
- 1 banana
- 1 scoop organic vanilla protein powder
- 2 celery stalks, chopped

Method

1 Rinse the kale well and remove any thick stalks.

2 Peel and roughly chop the pineapple.

3 Peel the banana and break into three pieces.

4 Add all the ingredients to the blender, making sure they do not go past the MAX line on your machine.

5 Blend until smooth.

CHEF'S NOTE
Use more coconut water if you prefer.

KALE & MANGO SMOOTHIE

Ingredients

GLOWING SKIN

- 1 handful kale
- ½ mango
- 2 stalks celery, chopped
- 1 tbsp fresh flat-leaf parsley
- Water

Method

1 Rinse the kale, celery and parsley.

2 Peel & stone the mango.

3 Add all the ingredients to the blender, making sure they do not go past the MAX line on your machine.

4 Blend until smooth.

CHEF'S NOTE
Vitamin A rich kale is excellent for skin and eyesight.

SPINACH & SWEET POTATO SMOOTHIE

SERVES 1

Ingredients

BETA CAROTENES

- 1 banana
- 1 handful spinach
- 1 small sweet potato (cooked)
- 300ml/10½floz unsweetened almond milk
- 1 celery stalk, chopped

Method

1 Rinse the spinach well and remove any thick stalks.

2 Peel the banana and break into three pieces.

3 Add all the ingredients to the blender, making sure they do not go past the MAX line on your machine.

4 Blend until smooth.

CHEF'S NOTE

Almond milk is high in vitamin E, which is essential to your skin's health.

AVOCADO & COCONUT SMOOTHIE

SERVES 1

Ingredients

- 300ml/10½ floz coconut water
- 1 handful spinach
- 2 kiwis
- ½ avocado
- 1 celery stalk, chopped

HEART HEALTHY

Method

1 Rinse the celery & spinach well. Remove any thick stalks.

2 Peel the kiwis and cut them in half. Peel & stone the avocado.

3 Add all the ingredients to the blender, making sure they do not go past the MAX line on your machine.

4 Blend until smooth.

CHEF'S NOTE

Avocados are rich in healthy fatty acids, vitamins and antioxidants that can improve your skin from the inside.

KALE, KIWI & CORIANDER SMOOTHIE

SERVES 1

Ingredients

DIETARY FIBRE

- 1 handful kale
- 2 kiwis
- 1 orange
- 2 tbsp fresh coriander
- 1 stalk celery, chopped
- Water

Method

1 Rinse the kale, coriander and celery. Remove any thick stalks from the kale.

2 Peel the kiwis and orange, de-seed the orange.

3 Add all the ingredients to the blender, making sure they do not go past the MAX line on your machine.

4 Blend until smooth.

CHEF'S NOTE
Kiwi contains several skin friendly nutrients including vitamin C, E and antioxidants.

COCONUT, APPLE & GINGER SMOOTHIE

Ingredients

- ½ romaine lettuce
- 1 celery stalk, chopped
- ½ apple
- ¼ cucumber

- ¼ avocado
- ½ lemon
- 2cm/1 inch piece peeled fresh ginger
- 250ml/8½floz coconut water

Method

1 Rinse the lettuce, celery, apple, cucumber and parsley.

2 Core the apple. Peel & stone the avocado. Peel & de-seed the lemon.

3 Add all the ingredients to the blender, making sure they do not go past the MAX line on your machine.

4 Blend until smooth.

CHEF'S NOTE

Ginger contains around forty antioxidant properties that prevent free radical damage and protect against aging.

WINTER GREEN SMOOTHIE

Ingredients

ANTIOXIDANT NUTRIENTS →

- 1 carrot
- ½ orange
- 1 handful spinach
- 4 broccoli florets
- 1 banana
- 1 apple
- 1 celery stalk, chopped

Method

1 Rinse the spinach, celery, broccoli & apple. Remove any thick stalks from the spinach.

2 Peel the orange and banana. Core the apple, peel & de-seed the orange.

3 Add all the ingredients to the blender, making sure they do not go past the MAX line on your machine.

4 Blend until smooth.

CHEF'S NOTE
The presence of dietary fibre, vitamins, minerals and antioxidants in broccoli are beneficial to skin.

MINT TEA BLAST

Ingredients

- 120ml/4floz chilled mint tea
- 1 handful baby spinach
- ½ romaine lettuce
- 5 fresh mint leaves
- 1 lemon
- 1 tsp honey
- 1 celery stalk, chopped

Method

1 Rinse the spinach, lettuce and mint.

2 Peel and de-seed the lemon.

3 Add all the ingredients to the blender, making sure they do not go past the MAX line on your machine.

4 Blend until smooth.

CHEF'S NOTE

Lettuce is a rich source of vitamin A. Vitamin A increases cell turnover which in turn helps to revitalise your skin.

KEFIR SPINACH BLAST

SERVES 1

Ingredients

PROBIOTIC GOODNESS →

- 1 handful baby spinach
- 2 celery stalks, chopped
- ½ avocado
- 1 kiwi
- 1 orange
- 120ml/4floz kefir
- Water

Method

1 Rinse the spinach & celery.

2 Peel and stone the avocado. Peel and de-seed the orange.

3 Halve, peel and stone the avocado.

4 Peel the kiwi.

5 Add all the ingredients to the blender, making sure they do not go past the MAX line on your machine.

6 Blend until smooth.

CHEF'S NOTE
Kefir contains lactic acid, an anti-aging ingredient.

CLEAN & GREEN SMOOTHIES

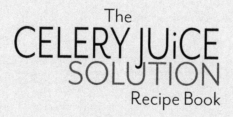

The
CELERY JUiCE
SOLUTION
Recipe Book

VEGETABLE & CITRUS BLAST

Ingredients

- 1 handful spinach
- ¼ cucumber
- 2 sticks of celery, chopped
- A few sprigs fresh parsley
- A few mint leaves
- 1 large carrot

- 1 apple
- 2 seedless orange segments
- 2 tbsp lime juice
- Water

Method

1 Rinse the ingredients well.

2 Remove any thick stalks from the spinach, core the apple and nip the ends off the carrot.

3 Add all the ingredients to the blender, making sure they do not go past the MAX line on your machine.

4 Blend until smooth.

CHEF'S NOTE

If you prefer a thinner drink, you might want to add more water after blending.

TROPICAL GREEN SMOOTHIE

Ingredients

- 2 handfuls spinach
- 175ml/6floz unsweetened almond milk
- ½ small banana
- 200g/7oz fresh pineapple,
- 2 pitted dates
- ½ - 1 tsp ground cinnamon
- 2 sticks of celery, chopped

Method

1 Rinse the spinach and remove any thick stalks.

2 Peel the banana and pineapple.

3 Halve and pit the dates

4 Add all the ingredients to the blender, making sure they do not go past the MAX line on your machine.

5 Blend until smooth.

CHEF'S NOTE
Use as much almond milk as you need to fill to the max.

FRUIT & LEAVES

Ingredients

- 1 romaine lettuce
- 3 sticks celery
- 1 handful spinach
- 1 apple

- 1 pear
- 1 banana
- 1 tbsp lemon juice
- Water

Method

1 Rinse the ingredients well. Snap the celery and remove any thick stalks from the spinach.

2 Core the apple and pear, but don't peel them. Peel the banana and break into three.

3 Add all the ingredients to the blender, making sure they do not go past the MAX line on your machine.

4 Blend until smooth.

CHEF'S NOTE
Add coriander and parsley for extra health benefits and flavour!

PAPAYA SMOOTHIE

Ingredients

GREEN POWER

- 150g/5oz papaya
- 1 handful kale
- 1 handful spinach
- ½ banana
- ½ green apple
- 4 tbsp water
- 1 celery stalk, chopped

Method

1 Rinse the spinach, celery, kale and apple.

2 Peel the papaya and the banana; break the banana into three pieces.

3 Core the apple and cut the half in two.

4 Add all the ingredients to the blender, making sure they do not go past the MAX line on your machine.

5 Blend until smooth.

CHEF'S NOTE

If the mixture is too thick for your taste, add water and re-blend, making sure to stay below the MAX line.

MANGO & COCONUT SMOOTHIE

Ingredients

PROTECTS HEALTH

- 1 mango
- ½ lime
- ½ banana
- 2 handfuls kale
- 200ml/7floz light coconut milk
- 1 celery stalk, chopped

Method

1 Rinse the ingredients well.

2 Remove any thick stalks from the kale.

3 Add the coconut milk to the blender.

4 Peel and stone the mango. Peel and de-seed the lime. Peel the banana and break into three pieces.

5 Add all the ingredients to the blender, making sure they do not go past the MAX line on your machine.

6 Blend until smooth.

CHEF'S NOTE
Try with spinach or other chard instead of kale.

ORANGE & SWEET POTATO SMOOTHIE

Ingredients

INCREASES ENERGY

- 1 orange
- 100g/3½oz cooked sweet potato
- 3 handfuls kale
- 2 tbsp chia seeds
- 1 celery stalk, chopped

Method

1 Rinse the kale and remove any thick stalks.

2 Peel and de-seed the orange.

3 Add all the ingredients to the blender, making sure they do not go past the MAX line on your machine.

4 Blend until smooth.

CHEF'S NOTE
Sweet potatoes are a good source of potassium, dietary fibre & niacin.

STRAWBERRY & BASIL SMOOTHIE

Ingredients

STRESS BUSTER

- Handful strawberries
- Handful fresh basil leaves
- 1 tbsp chia seeds
- 1 banana
- 2 handfuls spinach
- 200ml/7floz almond milk
- 1 celery stalk, chopped

Method

1 Pour the almond milk into the blender.

2 Wash the strawberries, celery, basil and spinach.

3 Peel the banana and break into three pieces.

4 Add all the ingredients to the blender, making sure they do not go past the MAX line on your machine.

5 Blend until smooth.

CHEF'S NOTE
Basil is an excellent source of vitamin K and manganese.

GRAPE & SPINACH BLAST

Ingredients

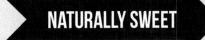

- 1 handful seedless green grapes
- 100g/3½oz pineapple
- 2 handfuls spinach
- ½ banana
- 2 celery stalks, chopped

Method

1 Rinse the grapes, celery and the spinach well.

2 Peel the pineapple & banana. Add to the blender along with all the other ingredients, making sure they do not go past the MAX line on your machine.

3 Blend until smooth.

CHEF'S NOTE
Experiment using quantities of water and ice to make your smoothie the consistency you like best.

VERY GREEN SMOOTHIE

SERVES 1

Ingredients

GREEN GOODNESS

- 2 handfuls kale
- ½ cucumber
- 3 celery stalks, chopped
- ½ lemon or lime
- 1 apple

Method

1 Rinse the ingredients well. Remove any thick stalks from the kale.

2 Core the apple.

3 Add all the ingredients to the blender, making sure they do not go past the MAX line on your machine.

4 Blend until smooth.

CHEF'S NOTE
Try a little fresh ginger blended with the smoothie to add a kick!

MOJITO SMOOTHIE

Ingredients

AIDS DIGESTION

- 1 handful spinach
- 6 fresh mint leaves
- 200ml/7floz coconut water
- 3 tbsp lime juice
- 1 banana
- 2 celery stalks, chopped

Method

1 Rinse the spinach, celery and mint well.

2 Peel the banana and break into three pieces.

3 Add all the ingredients to the blender, making sure they do not go past the MAX line on your machine.

4 Blend until smooth.

CHEF'S NOTE
If you have a sweet tooth, add a teaspoon of organic honey or agave nectar before blending.

ALMOND & STRAWBERRY SMOOTHIE

SERVES 1

Ingredients

- 1 handful spinach
- 1 handful kale
- 3 sprigs fresh parsley
- 1 handful strawberries
- 1 tbsp fresh lemon juice
- 1 celery stalk, chopped
- 200ml/7floz unsweetened almond milk

Method

1 Rinse the ingredients well.

2 Remove any thick stalks from the spinach & kale.

3 Add all the ingredients to the blender, making sure they do not go past the MAX line on your machine.

4 Blend until smooth.

CHEF'S NOTE

Almond milk is low in fat, but high in energy, proteins, lipids and fibre. It also contains calcium, iron, magnesium, phosphorus, potassium, sodium, and zinc.

WHEATGRASS POWER SMOOTHIE

Ingredients

- 1 banana
- ½ grapefruit
- ¼ avocado
- 1 handful each kale & spinach
- 1-inch peeled fresh root ginger
- 1 tsp wheatgrass powder
- 1 celery stalk, chopped

Method

1 Rinse the kale, celery and spinach well and remove any thick stalks.

2 Peel and de-seed the grapefruit. Peel and stone the avocado. Peel the banana and break into three pieces.

3 Add all the ingredients to the blender, making sure they do not go past the MAX line on your machine.

4 Blend until smooth.

CHEF'S NOTE
Referred to as a 'fountain of youth', wheatgrass has outstanding nutritional values and is packed with vitamins, minerals, amino acids and enzymes.

GOJI & CACAO SMOOTHIE

SERVES 1

Ingredients

- 250ml/8½floz coconut water
- 40g/1½oz avocado
- 3 tbsp low fat natural yogurt
- 100g/3½oz strawberries
- 1 tbsp goji berries

- 1 tbsp cacao powder
- ¼ tsp cinnamon
- A pinch of sea salt
- 1 tsp coconut oil
- 2 celery stalks, chopped

Method

1 Rinse the strawberries and remove the green tops

2 De-stone and peel the avocado..

3 Add all the ingredients to the blender, making sure they do not go past the MAX line on your machine.

4 Blend until smooth.

CHEF'S NOTE
Goji berries have higher levels of antioxidants than nearly all other superfoods – except cacao!

SUPERFOOD SMOOTHIES

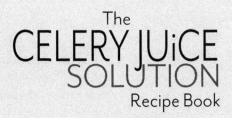

The
CELERY JUiCE
SOLUTION
Recipe Book

SWEET GOJI SMOOTHIE

Ingredients

- 1 tbsp dried goji berries
- 50g/2oz strawberries
- 1 tsp honey

- 250ml/8½floz unsweetened almond milk
- Water
- 2 celery stalks, chopped

Method

1 Soak the goji berries in a little water for around 15 minutes.

2 Rinse the strawberries well and remove the green tops.

3 Place all the berries in the blender. Add the honey, celery and almond milk to taste, making sure the ingredients do not go past the MAX line on your machine.

4 Top up with a little water if needed.

5 Blend until smooth.

CHEF'S NOTE
Goji berries are a wonderful superfood - they're packed with antioxidants, vitamins, minerals and fibre.

AVOCADO, BLUEBERRY & CHIA SMOOTHIE

Ingredients

- 75g/3oz avocado
- 50g/2oz fresh blueberries
- 1 tbsp chia seeds
- ¼ tsp cinnamon
- 2 tsp honey
- 2 celery stalks, chopped

Method

1 Rinse the blueberries well and place in the blender.

2 Peel and de-stone the avocado.

3 Add the chia seeds, cinnamon and honey.

4 Add water to the MAX line on your machine.

5 Blend until smooth.

CHEF'S NOTE

Chia seeds are fabulously rich in omega 3, protein and antioxidants.

KALE, COCONUT & PINEAPPLE SMOOTHIE

Ingredients

- 140g/4½oz kale
- 175ml/6floz coconut water
- 1 small banana
- 2 tbsp low fat natural yogurt

- 50g/2oz pineapple
- 2 tsp honey
- 2 celery stalks, chopped

Method

1 Rinse the kale well and remove any thick stalks.

2 Peel the banana and break into three pieces. Peel the pineapple.

3 Add all the ingredients the to the blender. Make sure they do not go past the MAX line on your machine.

4 Add a little water if needed to take it up to the MAX line.

5 Blend until smooth.

CHEF'S NOTE
Kale is believed to help prevent cardiovascular disease, several types of cancer, asthma, rheumatoid arthritis, and premature ageing of the skin.

GREEN TEA & MANGO SMOOTHIE

Ingredients

- 250ml/8½floz green tea (cooled)
- 150g/5oz mango
- 75g/3oz avocado
- 225g/8oz spinach
- A pinch of sea salt
- 1 tsp honey
- 1 celery stalk, chopped

Method

1 Make sure the green tea is no warmer than room temp.

2 Rinse the spinach well. Peel and de-stone the mango & avocado

3 Add all the ingredients the to the blender. Make sure they do not go past the MAX line on your machine.

4 Blend until smooth.

CHEF'S NOTE

The many nutrients found in avocados are thought to help protect your body from heart disease, cancer and degenerative eye disease.

MIGHTY BLUEBERRY FLAX SMOOTHIE

SERVES 1

Ingredients

- 125g/4oz blueberries
- 1 tbsp flax seeds
- 225g/8oz spinach
- 2 tbsp low fat Greek yogurt
- 100ml/3½floz coconut water
- 1 celery stalk, chopped

Method

1 Wash the spinach and blueberries well and place them in the blender.

2 Add the flax seeds, celery, yoghurt and coconut water. Make sure they don't go past the MAX line on your machine.

3 Top up with water as far as the MAX line.

4 Blend until smooth.

CHEF'S NOTE
Among many health benefits, flax seeds are believed to help lower blood pressure. They're also very rich in protein and fibre.

FRUIT CHIA SPICE SMOOTHIE

Ingredients

- 50g/2oz blueberries
- 6 tbsp low fat Greek yogurt
- 1 tbsp chia seeds
- ½ tsp ground cinnamon
- 2 tsp honey
- 2 celery stalks, chopped

Method

1 Rinse the blueberries and celery well.

2 Add them to the blender, along with the yoghurt, chia seeds, cinnamon and honey. Make sure they don't go past the MAX line on your machine.

3 Top up with water as far as the MAX line.

4 Blend until smooth.

CHEF'S NOTE

Cinnamon has been used throughout the ages to treat everything from a common cold to muscle spasms.

PEAR GREEN TEA

Ingredients

- 175ml/6floz strong green tea, chilled
- Pinch cayenne pepper
- ½ lemon
- 2 tsp agave nectar
- 150g/5oz pear
- 2 tbsp low fat plain yogurt
- 1 celery stalk, chopped

Method

1 Rinse, core and quarter the pear, leaving the skin on.

2 Peel and de-seed the lemon.

3 Add all the ingredients the to the blender. Make sure they do not go past the MAX line on your machine.

4 Blend until smooth.

CHEF'S NOTE
Green tea is packed full of antioxidants to help fight against cancer, anxiety and fat. It's also good for heart and brain health and promotes oral hygiene.

ZIPPY BERRY & BANANA SMOOTHIE

Ingredients

- 100g/3½oz mixed berries
- ½ small banana
- 225g/8oz spinach
- 1 tbsp coconut oil
- ¼ tsp cayenne pepper (or more to suit your own taste)
- 1 celery stalk, chopped

Method

1 Wash the berries and the spinach well.

2 Peel banana and add to the cup along with the coconut oil and cayenne pepper.

3 Add all the ingredients the to the blender. Make sure they do not go past the MAX line on your machine.

4 Add a little water if needed to take it up to the MAX line.

5 Blend until smooth.

CHEF'S NOTE

Spinach is a superfood well known for its nutrients and health benefits to bones, eyes & digestion. It's also extremely good for the complexion!

CHERRY BERRY HEMP BLEND

Ingredients

- 1 small banana
- 125g/4oz cherries, pitted
- 120ml/4floz unsweetened almond milk
- 50g/2oz raspberries
- 1 tbsp hemp seeds
- 1 celery stalk, chopped

Method

1 Rinse the cherries, raspberries and celery.

2 Place the pitted cherries in the blender.

3 Peel the banana, break it into 3 pieces and add.

4 Add the hemp seeds and almond milk making sure the ingredients do not go past the MAX line on your machine.

5 Blend until smooth.

CHEF'S NOTE

Hemp seeds have a great mixture of omega 3 and omega 6 fatty acids, most important for overall health. They also contain all 20 amino acids, including the essential ones that our bodies can't produce alone.

CACAO SUPERFOOD SMOOTHIE

Ingredients

- 250ml/8½floz coconut water
- 50g/2oz avocado
- 50g/2oz raspberries
- 1 tbsp cacao powder
- ½ tsp vanilla extract
- 225g/8oz spinach
- 1 celery stalk, chopped

Method

1 Rinse the raspberries and spinach well.

2 Peel and de-stone the avocado.

3 Add all the ingredients the to the blender. Make sure they do not go past the MAX line on your machine.

4 Add a little water if needed to take it up to the MAX line.

5 Blend until smooth.

CHEF'S NOTE

Raw cacao contains nearly four times the antioxidant content of processed dark chocolate.

KALE & CRANBERRY BLAST

Ingredients

- 225g/8oz fresh kale
- 100g/3½oz fresh cranberries
- 140g/4½oz orange

- 1 small banana
- 1 tbsp lime juice
- 1 celery stalk, chopped

Method

1 Rinse the kale, celery and cranberries. Remove any thick stalks from the kale.

2 Peel and de-seed the orange. Peel the banana and break into three.

3 Add all the ingredients the to the blender. Make sure they do not go past the MAX line on your machine.

4 Blend until smooth.

CHEF'S NOTE
Cranberries help prevent infections due to their high concentration of proanthocyanidins. They're also high in fibre, vitamin C and manganese.

Printed in Great Britain
by Amazon

80588506R00059